Let It Settle

Moving You from Anxiety and Chaos to Calm (Teens)

Epris E. Ezekiel

Contents

Understanding anxiety in children and teenagers.

Almost one-third of youngsters suffer from an anxiety disorder. Teens may suffer from a variety of anxiety disorders, including generalized anxiety, social anxiety, and panic disorder. Worry causes severe impairment in nearly 10% of teenagers, which means they cannot enjoy their normal lives or do day-to-day duties owing to the severity of their worry.

As parents, we always want the best for our kids. We want children to be healthy, happy, and resilient as they encounter life's obstacles. This is frequently easier said than done while dealing with daily pressures and parenting obligations. Anxiety is a prevalent problem in children, adolescents, and teenagers, occurring at various stages of development. Anxiety disorders can be diagnosed in children as young as four to eight years old, and a recent survey indicated that over 32% of adolescents in the United States had an anxiety condition. This figure has significantly increased over time. The study also found that one in every four to five teens suffers from a significant handicap as a result of their anxiety illness.

The COVID-19 epidemic has increased anxiety in children and teenagers due to interruptions in their typical school, family, and peer interactions. It is not always easy to distinguish between typical anxieties and anxiety disorders in children and adolescents, especially during these stressful times. For example, young people frequently worry about their homework or upcoming examinations, although this is usually just transitory once the current stressor has passed. However, if a child's anxiety becomes excessive and interferes with their everyday functioning, it can have a severe impact on their overall quality of life.

While dealing with your child's anxiety can be stressful, there is good news: anxiety is a very treatable disorder. You can also do a lot to aid your child. Rather than assuming that your child will outgrow their anxiety, it is best to begin taking steps as soon as possible to help them deal with their symptoms and recover control of how they see the world around them.

If you're a teen dealing with anxiety issues, or a parent looking to link your adolescent with resources and treatment, we've identified some critical tactics you may employ to alleviate symptoms and seek help if they become too overwhelming.

Chapter 1

What is anxiety?

Anxiety is a common aspect of life that affects everyone. When anxiety becomes overwhelming and does not go away, it may indicate the presence of an anxiety disorder. Anxiety can be addressed with treatment and the support of family and friends. Anxiety affects both the body and the psyche. Your teenager may frequently feel tight, restless, or irritated, and they may be concerned about their current circumstances or what will happen ahead. Anxiety is typical, especially among teenagers. It can boost motivation at school, sport, or job. However, if worried feelings persist, they might interfere with academic performance, social interaction, and enjoyment of life.

If your teenager's nervous sensations persist and appear out of proportion to the situation, they may have an anxiety disorder. Anxiety disorders are more than just excessive anxiety. It occurs when your teenager's anxieties and worries cause distress and prevent them from doing what they want or should be doing.

Anxiety symptoms differ between children and teenagers.

Anxiety symptoms vary greatly and are frequently left untreated in children and teenagers. Anxiety disorders in children are distinguished by irritability, nervousness, excessive worrying, shyness, sleep disturbances, and/or physical symptoms such as headaches or digestive problems.

What happens in their environment has a significant impact on children. They may feel depleted and separated from others, as well as afraid or ashamed. Children with anxiety may struggle to make friends or participate in other social activities.

Some of the most prevalent symptoms in youngsters are:

- ✓ Complaining frequently about not feeling well
- ✓ Crying occurs frequently.
- ✓ Being tense or fidgeting.
- ✓ Having tantrums or rage problems.
- ✓ Sleep disturbances or nightmares
- ✓ Concentrating is difficult.

The majority of teens' worries are related to their self-image. These may include academic achievement and pressure to succeed in school, how others see them, and body image problems related to physical development.

Teens' anxiety is often hidden since they

tend to conceal their thoughts and feelings. Some of the indications to watch for are:

- ✓ Constantly seeking reassurance.
- ✓ Substance abuse.
- ✓ Sleep issues.
- ✓ Refusing to attend school.
- ✓ Difficulties at school or unexpected bad performance.
- ✓ Irritability or lashing out at others.
- ✓ Withdrawal from friendships and social activities.
- ✓ Constant fear or worry regarding everyday parts of their existence.

Anxiety, regardless of the precise symptoms your kid or teen exhibits, can have a severe impact on their thoughts, emotions, and physical health. As a result, their intellectual and social functioning may suffer. Helping individuals deal with the problem begins with identifying the sources of their anxiety symptoms.

Anxiety can affect anyone at any time. Anxiety is the most prevalent mental health disorder. It impacts millions of young people in the United States.

Anxiety disorders are characterized by excessive worry about daily events or activities (for example, work or homework) that occur regularly and interfere with one's educational, occupational, and/or social life.

Chapter 2

How common is anxiety among young people?

- ✓ Unfortunately, just 7% of young individuals in need of mental health care obtain it.
- ✓ According to research conducted by the National Research Council and the Institute of Medicine, around 32% of teenagers in the United States suffer from anxiety disorders.
- ✓ Anxiety disorders are more common in women than in men, although age, race, and geography have little bearing on who develops anxiety.

Anxiety is not all the same.

Anxiety is the body's typical stress response. Children suffering from clinical anxiety, on the other hand, have disruptions in their everyday social, academic, and family lives. Though anxiety is a common emotional experience, excessive anxiety can suggest an issue that must be addressed.

It might be difficult to tell what kind of anxiety someone is feeling. Some anxieties are temporary and situational, while others are sudden and irrational.

Understanding the differences between stress, worry, uncertainty, panic, and social anxiety might help you better understand someone's anxiety symptoms.

Fear vs. Anxiety

Fear is the emotional response to an actual or perceived threat. Anxiety is the anticipation of a potential threat. People also use the term "anxiety" to signify persistent nervousness or a constant feeling of tension or stress.

Stress and Anxiety

Stress and anxiety are both emotional responses. Stress is typically triggered by an external event, such as taking a test or getting into a quarrel with a friend. Anxiety, on the other hand, is an internally generated fear that appears to take on a life of its own.

Both have comparable symptoms, including exhaustion, difficulty focusing, anger or irritation, and trouble sleeping. Clinical anxiety, unlike stress, is not a temporary condition that goes away once the stressor is removed.

Uncertainty

Anxious people are less tolerant of uncertainty. Anxiety sufferers sometimes refer to this as "fear of the unknown."

Those who worry excessively associate uncertainty with negative results. People suffering from anxiety may try to limit the number of unclear circumstances they experience to reduce their likelihood of a future threat. This avoidance exacerbates anxiety in the long run.

Panic

A panic attack is a bout of worry that lasts between 10 and 30 minutes and is accompanied by at least a few physical symptoms, such as a racing heart or shortness of breath. Panic attacks can occur unexpectedly or in response to a specific stimulus.

People with panic disorder have unexpected panic episodes and are afraid of having them again. They may also begin to avoid circumstances in which they believe they might have a panic attack.

Individuals with panic disorder frequently feel as if they are losing control, suffering a heart attack, or about to die.

Some of the physical signs of panic disorder are:

- ✓ Stomach distress
- ✓ Dizziness
- ✓ Shortness of breath.
- ✓ Chest discomfort.
- ✓ Sweating
- ✓ A rapid heartbeat

Social Anxiety

Social anxiety disorder is defined as the dread of being evaluated or embarrassed in social circumstances. Children frequently experience social anxiety in peer contexts, including school and extracurricular activities. It may also happen while interacting with adults or others in positions of power.

The root of social anxiety in children and

adolescents is a fear of being judged adversely by others in social circumstances. Their anxiety could be that others perceive them as worried, weak, dumb, dull, scary, unclean, or unlikeable. Some children and teenagers are afraid of offending others and being rejected as a result. Children who have social anxiety may avoid a variety of social experiences, including attending class, eating in front of others, engaging in extracurricular activities, ordering in restaurants, using public restrooms, and attending social events with peers.

Some of the key signs of social anxiety include:

- ✓ Shrink back to make oneself less conspicuous.
- ✓ Clinging to a classmate or parent.
- ✓ Freezing in Place
- ✓ Cry or throw a tantrum.

- ✓ Staring
- ✓ Sweating
- ✓ Stammering and stuttering
- ✓ Trembling
- ✓ Blushing

Social anxiety results in significant avoidance of social encounters. Often, the person's strong fear and anxiety worsen as they avoid the scenario. Chronic social anxiety usually lasts at least six months. Before a diagnosis is made for social anxiety disorder, symptoms must last at least six months.

Separation anxiety often peaks at age three. As children's brain function develops, they become more aware that the absence of an attachment figure is not permanent. In addition, as kids become older, they become more independent.

However, in those with separation anxiety disorder, this fear does not go away and may even worsen.

Chapter 3

What You Don't Know About Anxiety

Although the term "anxiety" is widely used, it is still a poorly understood condition. To properly comprehend anxiety in children and adolescents, we must first define it. Here are some prevalent myths regarding anxiety.

Myth: People can just "snap out" of their anxiety.

Anxiety is not like a light switch that can be turned on or off. While a youngster or teen's anxiety about being around strangers or being in a tight place may appear inconsequential, it is not to them. Because the cycle of worry and avoidance perpetuates itself, most people with anxiety require professional assistance to break it.

Myth: Anxiety Is Not Treatable.

Anxiety is highly treatable. Every case of anxiety is as individual as the child or adolescent who is diagnosed with it. What works for one person may not work for another, therefore patience is required to identify the treatment and support needed to help each young person flourish.

Myth: People Need Medication to Manage Their Anxiety.

In many circumstances, anxiety can be treated without the need for long-term medication. Medication may be prescribed for a short period to alleviate symptoms as a patient begins treatment. There are numerous effective techniques to manage anxiety, including meditation and mindfulness programs, individual and group therapy, exercise, and others. Medication is only one option for treating anxiety, which may or may not be effective for the   patient.

Myth: Children aren't anxious; they're simply shy.

Shy children and teenagers may be more likely to experience social anxiety, but the two are not synonymous. Being shy does not induce excessive anxiety or terror when placed in a social setting. Shyness is also a personality trait in children. Social anxiety is a dread of shame in a social situation that leads to avoidance.

Myth: Children and teenagers don't have anxiety; they only want attention.
Anxiety manifests physically differently in various people. As a result, children and teenagers may get angry, irritable, sleep poorly, withdraw, or have tantrums. While these activities may draw attention, anxiety may be influencing their thoughts and actions,

prompting people to react. Understanding the myths surrounding anxiety is one of the first steps toward understanding the disease. The more we know about it, the more equipped we are to assist others in seeking a diagnosis and care without fear of criticism or stigma.

Causes of anxiety in teenagers

There are numerous reasons why children get worried. Anxiety disorders are most likely caused by a mix of environmental and physiological causes. Anxiety runs in families and is more common in females than males. Anxiety disorders cover a wide range of mental health difficulties, including generalized anxiety disorder (GAD), obsessive-compulsive disorder (OCD), panic disorder, post-traumatic stress disorder (PTSD), social anxiety disorder, and other particular phobias. Some children can experience separation anxiety, which includes fear and anguish over being away from home.

What Causes Anxiety in Children and Teens?

Several causes can contribute to anxiousness. Factors may be inherited, learned, environmental, or biological.

Biological

Neurotransmitters are molecules in the brain that communicate with our bodies about how we should feel. People may be physiologically predisposed to anxiety if neurotransmitters do not send the correct messages at the appropriate times.

Environmental

Anxiety might arise as a result of a traumatic event, such as loss, illness, repeated home or school changes, bullying, or abuse. Anxiety can also co-occur with depression, attention-deficit/hyperactivity disorder, autism spectrum disorders, eating disorders, and other mental health issues.

Learned

While some children are predisposed to anxiety, being around nervous adults might cause toddlers to replicate worried behaviors. After parents express fear of and avoidance of a circumstance or object, children may also exhibit anxiety toward it.

Genetic

Just as a child might inherit their parents' height, they can also acquire their parents' worry.

Chapter 4

Tips for Moving Teens from Anxiety to Calmness

Tip 1: Promote healthy social media use.

Because studies show positive and negative effects, talking with youngsters about the benefits and drawbacks of social media is a smart place to start.

Instead of merely forcing your child to put their phone away, which may only increase their worry, you can take more constructive steps:

- ✓ If social media is interfering with your

child's schooling, sleep, or participation in extracurricular activities, limit their screen time.

✓ Encourage your child to cut links with those who make unpleasant remarks about them, and remind them to be careful when making comments about others. Teens, in particular, can be impetuous and fail to comprehend that the stuff they are posting is harmful or unsuitable.

✓ Remind kids, especially, that the photos they see on social media are frequently digitally manipulated and do not accurately reflect real life. Similarly, articles about parties or events to which they were not invited are frequently edited to make them appear more enjoyable than they were.

✓ Set aside a time when the entire family is

free of screens, including phones and computers. This can be done daily for a short length of time, or over the weekend when you are busy with family activities.

✓ Encourage your child to spend more time with friends in person and engage in creative activities rather than focusing on the number of "likes" their social media posts receive. If screen time does not become a habit early on, youngsters will learn to entertain themselves in alternative ways.

✓ Set a good example for your youngster by restricting your personal screen time and use of social media.

Tip 2: promote healthy sleep hygiene. Because anxious children frequently have difficulty sleeping, developing a consistent and soothing sleep regimen is critical. Set a regular sleep pattern, limit exercise and light exposure near bedtime, and avoid caffeine.

Make sure your child is comfortable and safe before bedtime, with few distractions to aid in falling asleep. Their bedroom should be cool, peaceful, and inviting. Screen usage on computers, phones, televisions, and video games should be limited to at least one hour before bedtime. This is a great time to read to your child or listen to peaceful, soothing music. A younger child may feel more secure with a nightlight on or a plush animal or soft blanket to keep them company.

Tip 3: Be a positive role model for your youngster.

Your child looks up to you and wants you to show them how to deal with stress and worry. The way you deal with frustration and express rage is an excellent example. When faced with challenges or difficult situations, try to be as calm and patient as possible. The manner you speak and what you say can have a significant impact on even the most challenging teenager's values and conduct.

Parents who care for themselves by getting adequate sleep, exercising frequently, and eating a nutritious diet might inspire their children to do the same. If you practice yoga, meditation, or other relaxation techniques, your children are more likely to prioritize their well-being. Avoid making harsh comments about your own body, as this can lead to low self-esteem and body shaming.

Modeling a healthy lifestyle can teach your children crucial things. We all make errors, and children should see that, despite their imperfections, parents can overcome adversity.

This can assist relieve any unneeded stresses that may be contributing to your child's anxiousness.

Tip 4: Use relaxation techniques with your youngster.

Offer to practice deep breathing or meditation activities with your youngster. This will acknowledge how they are feeling and offer proactive relaxing techniques that you can attempt together. When children are worried, their breathing typically becomes shallow. You can have your child practice deep belly breathing by placing one hand on their chest and the other on their abdomen. When they inhale, their stomach should expand; when they exhale, it should contract.

Mindful breathing entails focusing on your breathing and paying attention to the current moment. Allow your youngster to close their eyes and breathe slowly in and out. They may examine their bodies for tense places while breathing. They can then picture a sense of warmth and comfort to alleviate their suffering in these regions.

Older children and teens may also enjoy trying out different types of yoga, meditation, guided imagery, and other relaxation techniques. Turning off cell phones and social media and focusing on their "happy place" is a valuable skill to practice every day. Your teen can recall a specific event or situation that makes them feel peaceful, secure, and satisfied. Perhaps this is related to spending time at the beach, a calm holiday destination, or being surrounded by nature. Visualization of beautiful visuals or pleasant sounds is an excellent technique to induce this state of calm.

Tip 5: Address their anxiety appropriately. This may seem obvious, but as a parent dealing with an anxious youngster, you must remain as calm and optimistic as possible. How you respond to your child's ideas and behaviors can have a big impact on their capacity to cope.

Develop your child's coping skills.

Instead of ignoring your child's anxiety triggers, you can help them build healthy coping mechanisms. Giving your child frequent positive feedback will help them feel more capable and confident. Set short, realistic, and achievable goals. When a goal is met, you can add, "I'm so proud of the way you handled the situation and worked through your anxiety."

Make it a point to praise your child's efforts whenever they demonstrate perseverance or tackle their concerns. If a setback occurs, encourage your youngster that it is a learning opportunity that will help them conquer future hurdles. Discuss with them what they could do differently next time to achieve a better result. They will feel more empowered as they take charge of the situation.

Be supportive but not controlling.

The trick is to assist your child manage their anxiety without becoming overprotective in an attempt to eliminate it. You are already providing a lot of support by listening carefully and exhibiting empathy.

You can also discuss how to handle various circumstances. If your youngster has separation anxiety and was at a friend's house and frightened about returning home, discuss appropriate replies. For example, your child may ask the friend's mother what time you'll be picking them up, or they could request that the mother phone you to find out when you'll be there. Having these methods in place can assist in reassuring your youngster and lessen worry.

Talk with your child about their concerns. Begin a conversation with your child by asking them to share their thoughts about their anxieties. Simply telling a child not to worry or stop thinking about their difficulties does not provide support or validation. It is best to tell your child that it is normal for them to be terrified, and to highlight that you will be there to help them every step of the way.

If your child is having difficulty expressing their feelings, ask them to do so through a tale. Stepping outside of themselves may help your child feel more at ease and better able to express their sensations and emotions.

Show compassion and understanding.

Expressing encouragement and compassion, paired with a collaborative approach to finding practical solutions, can be an effective technique. According to research, mother empathy has a major impact on reducing children's discomfort.

Let your child know that anxiety is nothing to be embarrassed by and that you are here to assist them in understanding what causes their anxiety and how to handle it. This collaboration method creates a shared link between you and your child while also improving your youngster's ability to manage anxiety.

Additional suggestions for assisting a teen

Many of the approaches listed above can help both children and teenagers with anxiety. However, because adolescents and teens frequently have some awareness of worry and anxiety disorders, some extra measures may be useful.

Talk with your teenager about anxiety. Reassure your teenager that worry can be a protective emotion in some situations. Anxiety makes us aware of potential threats and helps us stay safe. That unpleasant sensation in the belly that we sometimes get could be a hint of a potential threat. Feeling worried can serve a beneficial purpose since paying attention to these warning indicators allows you to avoid dangerous circumstances. You can also help your kid feel less scared of their anxiety by discussing what they can do to improve a certain circumstance in the future.

Maintain an open dialogue with your teenager. Maintaining successful contact with teenagers can be challenging and even uncomfortable at times. Teenagers will not always confide in their parents when they gain independence. A helpful communication approach will increase trust and comfort while communicating their feelings.

It is critical to have constant communication with teenagers and inquire about their day. They may not go into great detail, but they will understand that you are genuinely interested and concerned about them. A few words of encouragement can have a big impact. Tell your teen you are proud of them and their progress.

If they express concern or anxiety about a specific issue, this is a time to start a more in-depth discussion. Validate their sentiments by stating things such as, "I know this is a difficult situation" or "That sounds very hurtful."

Prepare to tackle challenging situations: Discuss sensible and irrational answers to your teen's issues, whether they are academic, social, or general. Recognize that certain situations can cause worry, but put them in context to prevent exaggerating these sensations and causing additional concern. Teenagers may consciously or unintentionally exaggerate their feelings of hurt or fear, and they may become argumentative if they believe you, as a parent, don't understand.

When discussing how they handled a situation,

suggest some alternate approaches that might be more beneficial. For example, if your kid earned a failing score on a test and reacted by describing themselves as stupid or believing they'll never graduate, you can assist them reframe their erroneous views. Help them see the problem in a more realistic light by highlighting that this is only one test and that they can improve their results by studying harder or working with a tutor.

Use active listening skills: Teenagers rely on their parents for emotional support and outlets. You can help them feel less anxious by listening attentively and validating their feelings without judgment or condemnation. You can accomplish this by giving your teen your entire attention, making eye contact to demonstrate that you are interested in what they are saying, and nodding sometimes to indicate that you are listening. Avoid interrupting your teen while they are speaking so that they feel free to express themselves fully.

Improve your teenager's self-esteem.

Instead of focusing on your teen's weaknesses, highlight his or her positives. Instead of focusing on their anxiety, highlight their positive characteristics. It might be as simple as congratulating your teen on their thoughtfulness, generosity, or concern for others. Your teen may also possess significant intellectual or character attributes that distinguish them as individuals. Instead of feeling like they don't belong, emphasize that their distinctiveness should be embraced.

- ✓ If your kid has a special interest or talent, such as art, music, or sports, you can use it to keep them motivated. Showing how proud you are and acknowledging the rewards of your dedication will bolster your confidence. Mastering any talent will increase self-esteem and redirect attention away from their worry. Remember, the goal is not to be perfect; rather, they should provide their best effort to succeed depending on their talents.

✓ Building resilience and self-confidence might help your kid identify their problem-solving abilities. If they perform well on an exam or school task, you can do more than just congratulate them. You can also remind them how much time they spend studying and preparing. This will demonstrate the importance of their efforts to achieve rather than constantly worrying about the outcome.

Be mindful of the expectations you create: Teens might frequently feel overwhelmed by high expectations and pressure to perform. Setting realistic goals will help guide kids toward academic success while reducing their anxiety about grades and test results.

Demonstrate the importance of assisting others: Participating in good activities that benefit others can increase a teen's self-esteem while also providing a beneficial, healthy distraction from anxiety. Encourage them to explore volunteer opportunities in the community for causes they care about. Joining a group or club with other teenagers who share their interests can also help them improve their social skills and feel more connected.

Chapter 5

What Are the Treatment Options for Anxiety?

There are several therapy options for anxiety disorders. Therapy, drugs, support groups, and proven stress management practices can all help people manage their anxiety disorder successfully.

Acceptance & Commitment Therapy

ACT is a behavioral therapy that blends self-acceptance and mindfulness with a commitment to change based on one's ideals. This promotes psychological flexibility, which means that regardless of the patient's worry, they can adapt and remain present in the moment.

In ACT, the patient commits to confronting worries rather than avoiding them, and the patient learns to embrace difficult situations.

Interpersonal Therapy

IPT, which is commonly used to treat depression, is a short-term treatment for anxiety. IPT teaches patients how to grasp their underlying interpersonal issues to express their feelings more effectively.

Changes in social contexts, conflict with loved ones, and academic difficulties are among the most common interpersonal concerns addressed. IPT can assist patients to improve their communication and interpersonal skills.

Medication

Doctors can prescribe a variety of drugs to alleviate anxiety. Antianxiety drugs alleviate symptoms associated with anxiety, panic attacks, excessive worry, or dread. Selective serotonin reuptake inhibitors, or SSRIs, are an evidence-based class of medication. They can alleviate anxiety symptoms and depression symptoms, which are frequently associated with anxiety disorders.

Therapy

Most anxiety treatments involve talk therapy, sometimes known as psychotherapy. Talk therapy is an effective way to treat people with a wide range of mental health issues, including anxiety. Sessions can be held alone, with parents or families, or in a group environment. Patients who work directly with a therapist can learn to control their anxiety symptoms more effectively.

During therapy sessions, established treatment procedures are applied. Evidence-based treatments for pediatric anxiety include cognitive behavior therapy (CBT) combined with exposure and response prevention therapy (ERP), acceptance and commitment therapy (ACT), and interpersonal therapy (IPT).

Cognitive Behavior Therapy Using Exposure and Response Prevention

Cognitive behavioral therapy combined with ERP is one of the most successful techniques for treating anxiety problems.

CBT is a type of talk therapy that teaches children about the relationships between their ideas, feelings, and behaviors, as well as how to manage them. With exposure and reaction prevention, people eventually face their concerns and understand that they are capable of handling difficult situations.

These therapies assist the patient in recognizing and changing their negative thought patterns.

CBT can also help with social skills, such as reducing social anxiety.

Support Groups

There are numerous support groups for persons suffering from anxiety disorders, both in-person and online.

To guarantee children's health and safety, it is recommended that a doctor make recommendations before participating in a self-help or support group.

Stress Management Techniques

Those suffering from anxiety problems require specific attention to stress management. Meditation and coping skills help people relax, which can improve the effectiveness of therapy.

Here are some coping skills and meditation techniques:

- ✓ Going to a doctor or therapist to discuss stress-reduction measures
- ✓ Talking and exchanging experiences with others.
- ✓ Learning about your triggers
- ✓ Acceptance
- ✓ Deep Breathing Exercises
- ✓ Healthy sleeping habits, which include reduced screen time before bed
- ✓ Exercise, such as yoga
- ✓ Eating good meals and restricting coffee consumption
- ✓ Taking time out of the day to relax

How is anxiety diagnosed?

Anxiety should be diagnosed by a competent, licensed practitioner, such as a psychiatrist or a pediatrician.

Depending on the symptoms, a healthcare professional may do normal lab testing during the initial evaluation to rule out other potential reasons. In some cases, x-rays, scans, or other imaging tests may be necessary. The provider may ask the child and/or parent(s) a series of questions from a standardized questionnaire or have them fill out a self-assessment of symptoms.

Anxiety may be diagnosed alongside other diseases, particularly GAD, which has a high rate of co-occurring conditions.

In some situations, significant depression, substance abuse, post-traumatic stress disorder, and obsessive-compulsive disorder may coexist. If this is the case, further testing and treatment may be necessary.

Conclusion

Fear, worry, and anxiety are natural parts of being human (in fact, they are necessary for our survival), but when they damage our well-being or disturb our daily lives and health, we require assistance. As parents, we must help our children understand and control their emotions, as well as recognize when they may want additional assistance.

Our fast-paced world is not conducive... I am convinced that most of the stress and anxiety in children's lives stems from hidden pressures and overzealous expectations of well-meaning parents and teachers.